Intermittent Fasting

Learn the Physical and Mental Benefits of Fasting; Build Muscle and Lose Fat while Increasing Productivity and Metabolism

Ryan Greene

Table of Contents

Introduction 1

Chapter One: What Happens When We Fast? 3

Chapter Two: The Physical Benefits 5

Chapter Three: The Mental Benefits 9

Chapter Four: Lifestyle Benefits..12

Chapter Five: Common Types of Fasting 15

Chapter Six: Exercising on a Fast 22

Chapter Seven: What to Avoid... 24

Chapter Eight: Common Misconceptions About Fasting........27

Chapter Nine: Fasting Around the World 32

Final Words... 34

Introduction

Congratulations on downloading this eBook on Intermittent Fasting! In it, you'll find a summary of the benefits of fasting, including the history and science behind limiting your caloric intake to certain parts of the day.

Intermittent fasting is not a "diet", as you'll learn, it's a strategy for managing your calorie intake, and fasting can suit a large number of personal goals. By reading this book, you will gain a strong command of the core concepts of fasting, and you will have all the information you need to take advantage of one of the strategies for Intermittent Fasting. Whether you are trying to lose weight, increase muscle mass, reduce your body fat or you're looking for the most efficient ways to provide your body the nutrients it needs, fasting is a compelling answer.

Where does fasting come from? Culturally, humans have been fasting for centuries. Major religions like Christianity, Islam, Buddhism and more have presented fasting as a productive way to access your spirituality and become closer to a higher power. For many years, fasting has been a trusted medicinal path to improved health and wellness. Recently, however, the cellular benefits of fasting have begun to see the light of popular health and wellness publications. Common myths and fears about fasting are being put to rest, in favour of the age-old wisdom of limiting our caloric intake to certain times of day.

Modern scientific breakthroughs are starting to identify the benefits of allowing our bodies to enter phases of fast that they would never enter in a cycle of eating three square meals per day. Evidence shows many benefits to fasting, like improved metabolism and weight loss, associated improvements in heart and brain health, mood and stress levels. By allowing our bodies to reach the fasting phase, we can take our minds off of food for longer stretches during the day to focus and be productive in other areas. We can even push our bodies to longer life spans, more free of degenerative and chronic illnesses.

Don't wait another day to learn the basics of this lifestyle. Don't delay the physical and mental benefits of controlling your food intake. Start learning the science behind a centuries-old practice of controlling your body and your mind.

Read this book today and start living the lifestyle your body is geared for!

Chapter One
What Happens When We Fast?

In this chapter you will learn about the basic concept of "Intermittent Fasting". You will get an introduction to the fasting

Fasting is not dieting. The science behind Intermittent Fasting, or "IF," comes not from the content of food being eaten, but the timing of consumption. Our bodies act very differently when they have eaten recently: our metabolisms change, our hormones change, even our brain chemistry is altered when food is being digested.

The use of fasting, as opposed to dieting, is a deliberate effort to introduce your body to a state of non-digestion, which it may rarely experience when you eat three meals per day. That's because a "fasted" state, meaning the condition of being without food and thus no longer actively digesting, only occurs 8-12 hours after your last meal. When we eat three meals per day, and snack before bed, our body may never actually enter the "fasted" state. We will spend our entire day, and much of our sleep cycle, processing food from our latest meal.

Some interesting things happen to our bodies and our brains during the fasted state, and Intermittent Fasting has an explicit goal of letting the body spend the appropriate amount of time in this state.

First of all, consider the origins of our digestive schedules. Our distant ancestors weren't accustomed to three square meals per day, snacks, and entire shelves of processed food. Living in the wild, regular "fasting" meant only that food didn't show up regularly. The human body is capable of surviving for many days without food (Gandhi fasted for three weeks), and in our early history, going without food for a few days would have been normal. As a result, our bodies have evolved not simply to survive these lean times, but to perform important functions during these different states of being fed. The chemical composition of our bodies changes when food is present, and our cells enter different regenerative states when food is gone.

The modern routine of eating regularly, constantly and without pause, prevents our bodies from entering these productive alternate states to which they have been accustomed for thousands of years.

That presents problems, because our bodies rarely enter these states of being "fasted" anymore. Consider personally, the last time you had nothing to eat for more than 12 hours. Such an occurrence is most likely rare, and probably a negative experience for most people. Part of Intermittent Fasting is adjusting our perception of going without food for longer periods, and to consider that such times can actually be positive for our health.

Culturally, we have built a significant amount of concern around skipping meals. We say things like "Never miss breakfast, it's the most important meal of the day!" We worry that being hungry will cripple our mood, make us ornery and unable to process new information. Snickers campaign called "You're Not You When You're Hungry" plays on our fear of being "hangry," a mix of hungry and angry.

The truth is that our bodies are built to withstand, even benefit from, short intervals of fasting. If we can learn to adjust our lifestyles to allow our bodies to experience productive fasts, there are many benefits available to us.

In this chapter you have learned that our bodies are accustomed to periods of what we call "fasting," and that during these times, our bodies undergo important processes that modern humans rarely get to take advantage of as a result of regular eating.

Chapter Two
The Physical Benefits

In this chapter you will learn what happens to your body when you fast, at the cellular level.

One of the major differences between being fed and being in the fasted state is the presence of higher amounts of insulin, the hormone released to process and access sugars in the food we eat. We need insulin to manage our blood sugar, so our bodies release insulin when we are digesting, to process all the new material and keep our blood sugar levels stable. When we fast, the level of insulin constantly present in the blood is lowered significantly, which has been shown to improve our insulin sensitivity. Insulin sensitivity is a measure of how much insulin is needed to maintain our blood sugar. For reference, diabetics have difficulty with insulin production and sensitivity, and use injections of insulin to supplement their body's natural creation of the hormone. Insulin also makes it difficult for the body to access and burn stored body fat. So, simply by allowing our bodies to access a fasted state more often, we can better utilize powerful hormones like insulin, and improve our body's ability to burn fat.

To understand in more detail how our bodies burn fat when fasting, it's important to understand how our bodies store energy. When we eat, we use insulin to transform our food into two primary types of stored energy that we can use later: sugar, and fat. These types of energy are stored in different ways in the liver, and that matters when it comes time to use them. Sugar is stored easily and simply, and our body's prefer to use sugar for energy because it is so easily accessible. Fat is more difficult to utilize as an energy source, because it is stored differently and requires additional chemical processes to access and use. Our modern behaviour of eating every few hours serves only to constantly replenish our stores of sugar, which our bodies then immediately turn around and use. We never give our bodies the opportunity to access and use stores of fat for the production of energy. Instead we live from meal to meal, focused only on giving our body new access to easy-to-use sugar based energy. Once we enter the fasted state, our bodies only then begin to leverage fat stores. This process of changing energy sources really kicks in at about 24 hours. Keep that in mind as you learn about the different fasting protocols, which manage your tolerance up to about 24 hours of fasting.

When your body gets better at managing blood sugar, and reduces these stores of fat, it also is able to maintain better heart health. Intermittent Fasting has been shown in this way to help overall cardiac health by reducing cholesterol, reducing fat content, and improving blood sugar levels. Fasting may also help reduce major causes of inflammation in our bodies. Inflammation is a contributor to many potential chronic health problems.

Another major hormonal change that occurs between the "fed" state and the "fasted" state is the production of the Human Growth Hormone. You've probably heard about HGH in professional sports drug scandals before. Players found guilty of abusing HGH are taking doses of the hormone to supplement their body's production. All they had to do to take advantage of up to five times the normal production of HGH was fast! That's right, our bodies being to release the Human Growth Hormone in large amounts once our bodies have entered the fasting state.

Similar to the release and production of more Human Growth Hormone, entering a fasted state also stimulates production of the hormone Testosterone, which can be beneficial for both men and women. Testosterone is a useful hormone for an increase of the body's metabolism, and is an active ingredient in creating more muscle.

Not surprisingly, when your body enters the fasted state, it also begins to look toward your stored fats for sustenance. This is one of the only times your body releases certain hormones in order to target these fat stores. For this reason, fasting is a compelling weight-loss tool for people with good diets and regular exercise. It's important to understand that this happens 12 hours after our last meal, no matter how big that meal was. That's why fasting is less of a diet plan, and more of a calorie consumption strategy. Even if you ate the same number of calories as last week, but this week you limited the intake of those calories to be within a small window of time each day, then you would still allow your body to enter the fast state each day.

Finally, our bodies behave differently at the cellular level when we enter the fasted state, 12 hours after our last meal. Autophagy is the process by which our cells undergo a controlled breakdown of unnecessary proteins. Think of this like a crucial cellular "trash removal," which occurs most effectively during periods of fasting. This interesting cellular change is why some scientists believe that Intermittent Fasting is useful in preventing many types of cancer.

This process if accelerated autophagy is very interesting, not just for the prevention of cancer, but for the overall prolonging of life. Our bodies' ability to remove excess cellular material and regenerate critical cellular structures is the key to living longer, healthier lives. One study from the 50s followed 120 seniors, half of which fasted every other day. The sixty seniors who practiced Intermittent Fasting spent 123 days in the hospital, and 6 passed away. Of the 60 seniors who did not fast, there were almost double the deaths and number of days in hospital. This could point to the benefits of inspiring our body's natural autophagic processes as a method of prolonging our healthy lives.

Put these bodily changes into perspective. Remember that our bodies were originally intended to help us survive periods of famine, and take advantage of periodic feasts. When our production of hormones like Human Growth Hormone, Testosterone, Insulin and certain fat-burning hormones changes as a result of not having food, our bodies are responding in a way that benefits us. These hormones are producing energy for us to use, muscle for us to use, and are asking our bodies to grow and become stronger in order to find the next food store. We begin discarding unnecessary cellular material and converting it to energy through autophagy. These are all changes that our bodies aren't used to experiencing, important state changes that we can derive many benefits from if we allow ourselves to experience some surface level discomfort during an adjustment period to intermittent fasting.

In this chapter, you learned about the chemical and cellular changes our bodies undergo when fasting. You learned that these changes, often rarely experienced in our modern culture, can afford compelling physical benefits like the weight loss, blood sugar regulation, and the prevention of cellular deterioration. In the next chapter, you will learn about the mental benefits of fasting.

Chapter Three
The Mental Benefits

In this chapter you will learn what is theorized to happens inside your brain when you enter a fasted state. Just as our bodies change their chemical and cellular processes to meet the condition of being hungry, our brains change in kind.

This is described by some scientists as a "mild state of stress," which for the purposes of our body and mind, serves to keep us sharp and reduce waste. The neurological equivalent of autophagy has to do with a protein called Brain-Derived Neurotrophic Factor, or BDNF. The role of these proteins are to prevent stressed neurons in our brain from simply dying off. This protein works to keep as many neurons as it can, which is important for us because neurons are the foundational cells of our brain's network! Neurologists study the presence of BDNF in patients with Alzheimer's, for example. One study found that when rats fast, the levels of BDNF in their brains are increased, which means that their brains are working harder to retain usable neurons.

So why should we introduce more stress to our body systems? Don't we have enough stress in our lives already? Certainly experience stress, but by pushing our bodies with Intermittent Fasting we can take advantage of another mental benefit: reduction of stress. This might seem counterintuitive, since Fasting is a "mild" form of stress. Actually, what we are doing is exchanging a more dangerous form of stress for this new "mild" version. Today, we put an undue stress on all of our body processes, by feeding our bodies constantly. We are facilitating bodily processes that aren't natural. We continually provide our bodies with fat to store that we will rarely ever use again. We ask our body constantly to store and use the sugar based energy called Glycogen, instead of exercising our body's natural instinct to dip occasionally into fat stores for energy. This places additional stress on our bodies by negatively producing cholesterol, placing extra burden on our cardiovascular system. Our blood pressure rises, blood sugar levels become more difficult to manage, and for these reasons we see the increased incidence of chronic conditions like diabetes and heart disorders. These are states of increased stress that our bodies are forced to manage over the course of years of mistreatment through overeating. Intermittent Fasting is a strategy that encourages our body's natural response to a once common condition of scarce food availability, which again is a "mild" form of stress. This type of condition focuses us, makes our body more efficient, and helps us manage the more stressful conditions of high blood pressure and volatility in our blood sugars.

Imagine again, for context, that your brain chemistry is designed to help you survive stressful situations without food and give you the mental capacity you need to plan and strategize. The increased presence of this special type of protein during times of fasting makes sense as a special strategy your brain employs to keep you sharp and alert.

The opposite scenario is also helpful in understanding our body's responses to fasting. If our biological purpose is to find and consume food, so that we can procreate, then our body needs to be at it's most focused, finely tuned, and prepared for maximum effort when it is decidedly without food. When our body's have been completely satisfied, and by evolutionary standards three square meals per day certainly qualifies, then our body may feel capable of letting down its guard and settling into a comfortable routine. It no longer needs to employ generations of chemical and mechanical responses to perceived needs, a certain amount of which can actually yield important benefits for us today.

So what is happening when we get angry as we get hungry today? Our bodies are accustomed to eating regularly, and using insulin to manage a certain blood sugar all day. Any change to the schedule of our food is bound to incur some amount of irritability. The important thing to understand is that this is not a permanent state, and that the long term benefits of experiencing a fasted state regularly may include the prevention of certain conditions like Alzheimer's, through the production of proteins like BDNF.

The truth behind hunger and brain chemistry is that it takes a long time to incur the negative effects of hunger on our cognitive processing. Studies that compare the mental acuity of someone who has just eaten to someone who hasn't for 24 hours, even for 48 hours, find no compromised cognitive ability. The truth is that hunger doesn't begin to impair our focus for days, meanwhile the positive effects of Intermittent Fasting occur when we enter the fasted stage after only 12 hours.

In this chapter you have learned a little more about what happens to the brain when it enters the fasted state. You learned about Brain-Derived Neurotrophic Factors, which work to preserve neurons in your brain over time and can prevent neurological diseases like Alzheimer's. In the next chapter you will learn about the lifestyle benefits of Intermittent Fasting.

Chapter Four
Lifestyle Benefits

In this chapter you will learn how intermittent fasting can have an effect on the life you lead, including what you're capable of and how your attitude can change.

The first, most obvious benefit is the reduction of effort necessary in planning meals and cooking. This might seem simple, but it's an easy way to gain back some time and money each day that would otherwise be spent on preparing and eating food. As you'll see in the example fasting plans of later chapters, this can be one to two meals each day, which can amount to significant gains in money and time.

Eating healthy can be more difficult in many cases than eating poorly. Fast food is readily available, and eating healthy can demand more preparation, time, and money. Consider that by fasting, and removing a significant number of the instances in which you have to eat healthy, then it can be easier to eat healthy by focusing on meals like Lunch and Dinner.

Another benefit of fasting is the joy of eating! When food is reduced to a regular chore, then it can become boring as it becomes our master. By eating less, and affording ourselves more time (and money) to focus on those meals, we can actually spend more time enjoying the food we eat. Instead of counting calories all day, we can be free to revel in the tastes and experiences of the meals we do eat.

We spend a lot of our time each day thinking about food, acting on those thoughts, then managing the after-effects of having eaten. We wake up thinking about breakfast, we are planning lunch as shortly after we arrive at work, then we deal with the consequences of having a heavy lunch, or the hunger from having a light lunch, then we have larger dinners once we get home. So much of our lives revolve around food, the only other larger component of our lives is sleep! Imagine being able to focus (and be more focused) on the parts of our lives that aren't sleep or food.

A major part of this lifestyle change is a better understanding of what we think of as "hunger." When you fast, you start to truly come to grips with your body's urges. You realize that what you thought was "hunger" last week was closer to a simple memory of food, complete with a sensory experience, that made you remember what it was like to eat. That alone would have been enough to qualify in your brain as "hunger." The truth about hunger is that it's more significant when it's real. Your body begins to really ask you, out loud and with conviction, for food that it wants. Simply being able to discern between a reflex to eat and a sincere need to eat is an important benefit for your health. After fasting, you'll be at less risk of eating out of boredom, because you are more in touch with your body's needs.

The other side of this understanding of hunger is an overall reduction in calorie intake. Intermittent Fasting does not specifically prescribe a reduction in calories, but most participants do not completely compensate for the skipped calories and make up for them during the eating period. For example, during alternating day fasts, a participant eats nothing on one day, and does not automatically eat double the next day to make up for lost calories on day one. Instead, it's more common for the person to eat only slightly more than normal on the second day. Many of the benefits to health and wellness can also have roots in this inherent calorie deficit, present when fasting regularly.

To understand the differences in mood, focus, and motivation that are possible with Intermittent Fasting, remember again the evolutionary origins of these bodily processes. As a species, we historically have had to perform our absolute best during times of need, scarcity. We experience our most relaxed, lethargic selves when we have achieved our evolutionary goals of eating food (remember that 'food coma' from last Thanksgiving?)

Our bodies, by experiencing the fasted state every so often, start to regenerate through autophagy, and our bodies are retaining more neurons. Many people as a result report increased energy, focus, and vitality when they've adjusted to an Intermittent Fast that makes sense for them and their routine.

By introducing our bodies to just a small reminder of that past experience of small fasting intervals, we can reap some of the benefits our bodies developed over many generations of gene selection and evolution.

We can experience increased focus, mental acuity, and drive, simply by skipping breakfast several times per week. We can enjoy increased metabolism, and the associated fat-burning characteristics. All these benefits for free (not eating doesn't cost anything). You will also have more time on your hands as you will not be spending as much time eating or preparing meals.

These things alone can improve our mood, and as you'll learn from the chapter on Common Misconceptions, hunger doesn't have to be the overriding element to Intermittent Fasting.

In this chapter you have learned that you can expect certain improvements to your overall lifestyle by incorporating even the occasional fast into your schedule. In the next chapters, you will learn about some of the basic fasts you can start to take advantage of immediately!

Chapter Five
Common Types of Fasting

I n this chapter you will learn about one of the most common types of Intermittent Fasts. There are many ways to fast, but the characteristics of these fasts are all very similar. The key is to find the fast that works best for you, the fast that is attainable and repeatable, so that you can begin to enjoy the benefits of a regular fasted state.

Make sure to follow up your reading of this chapter with subsequent chapters on "what to avoid," and "common misconceptions." These will help balance your understanding of Intermittent Fasting and provide the safest way for you to get started if you so choose.

The 14/10 Fast

One of the most common Intermittent Fasts is what's known as the 14/10. This shorthand refers to the hours spent fasting(14) and the hours which can be spent eating (10). Recall that all that is needed for your body to enter a fasted state is 12 hours, which is most easily attained when done over the course of an evening, when sleep can be used to your advantage.

If you eat dinner each night at 7, and finish by 7:30, then by 7:30AM your body has entered a fast state, and has begun to increase production of important hormones and neurological proteins. It has ceased to focus on digesting the food from dinner, and is now getting to work making you stronger and more alert to find your next meal.

The 14/10 Fast asks you simply to delay your first meal of the day until at least 9:30AM, to give your body at least two hours in the fast state before again introducing a large meal to your system. For the next ten hours, until 7:30 PM, you can consume food normally. That's right, normally! Remember that Intermittent Fasting isn't a "diet," in that it doesn't regulate how much you eat and what you eat, it regulates when you eat. Simply by limiting your food intake to specific hours of the day, in order to allow your body to enter the fast state more often, you can experience weight loss, even if you eat a normal calorie load during those hours.

The 14/10 is a relatively easy way to introduce your body to the fast state without experiencing hunger pangs for large portions of the day. It is the recommended first step in phasing your Intermittent Fasting into your schedule. Try going three days on the 14/10 schedule, and see how you feel. You should experience a decrease in hunger by 9:30 AM on the third day.

The 16/8 Fast

The 16/8 fasting routine is classic. Once your body has adjusted to a 14/10 Fast, the 16/8 is the next step. This fast effectively skips breakfast every day, and asks you to resume your caloric intake at lunch. In our example, you finish eating a large dinner at 7:30 PM, and you would enter the fast state by 7:30 AM the next day. This time, instead of eating a late breakfast, you will ask your body to forego breakfast and remain in the fast state for four hours, until at least 11:30 AM. At this point you can eat normally until 7:30 PM, when you should finish dinner and major eating.

The 16/8 Fast is often somewhat familiar to people who don't naturally crave breakfast and usually wait until lunch to have anything substantial. This instinct to forego breakfast has been scorned, because we've all heard that "breakfast is the most important meal of the day." Skipping breakfast is also the easiest way to achieve longer daily fasts, since it's right on the heels of your sleep cycle.

Meal Skipping

With Intermittent Fasting, your goal is to allow your body to experience the fast state. Remember that it usually takes your body about 3 hours to digest your food, and a full 12 hours to enter the fast state. Skipping a meal when you aren't hungry is a great way to further acclimate your body to longer intervals of not eating. If you've started fasting by delaying your breakfast, and have eventually begun to skip breakfast entirely, don't feel pressured to eat lunch as soon as your fast interval is over. Use your morning to focus on your work, your task-list, your errands, even on working out. Occupy yourself, and take advantage of your body's lean focus and energy as it enters the fast state. If you come to lunch at say, noon, and you're still focused on the task at hand, use that energy to carry your fast a little longer. If you don't crave lunch at that point, skip it and plan on eating a big dinner.

Alternate Day Fasting

In the 1950's study of senior citizens doing Intermittent Fasts, the program called for some moderate fasting, like the 16/8 program, only every other day. This is another good way to acclimate your body to the fasting regimen. Try to start by delaying breakfast only every other day, as you gradually introduce the 14/10 and the 16/8 fast to your routine.

Consistency over the long term is a potential benefit of the Alternate Day Fasting regimen. By focusing one day on the fast, then allowing your body and brain to return to normal eating habits, you are able to stay more grounded and confident in your ability to participate in the alternating fasts.

24 Hour Fasts

These fasts are where people start to really get antsy. Few people remember the last time they went 24 hours without food. It may be one thing to skip breakfast, but it's quite another to skip three meals in a row. Our perception is that we will be drastically impaired, angry, almost feral. The truth is that cognitive ability isn't impaired due to calorie deprivation for several days. The perceived degradation is usually mental. We have trained ourselves to crave food every few hours, in the form of complete meals with multiple courses. Our bodies need to learn to forego these food extravaganzas if we are to take advantage of the benefits of the fast state.

The key is to make incremental progress in achieving a 24 hour fast. You shouldn't put this book down right now in order to stop eating for the next 24 hours.

Start by acclimating your body to the fast state one to two hours at time, by introducing the 14/10 and the 16/8 fasts.

A 24 hour fast is usually recommended only about once or twice per week, and is easier than you might think. In our example, you're eating dinner each night at 7PM, and finishing by about 7:30PM. In order to complete a 24 hour fast, you simply won't eat anything until the next dinner rolls around at 7PM.

Eat-Stop-Eat

This modification of Alternate Day Fasting suggests that you fast entirely for 24 hours, then eat without restriction for 24 hours, then return to the 24 hour fast. The idea is that if you limit your intake for one day, you won't double your intake the next day to make up for it. Most people will eat only slightly more than normal the next day, which results in a significant calorie deficit over the course of the week. That method of fasting, feasting, fasting can be difficult for many people to manage consistently and over long periods of time.

The 5:2 Diet (A version of Eat-Stop-Eat)

There is another popular version of Eat-Stop-Eat that focus on two back to back days of reduced calorie intake, with five otherwise normal intake days. During the "Fast" days, you can start by allowing yourself 500-600 calories during a fixed four hour eating window. This restricted eating method is one of the only times you will see an Intermittent Fast prescribe what or how much to eat during a "feasting" window. The 500-600 calories is often helpful for people who like the alternating plan, but can't manage 24 hour fasts so close in succession. This method helps them stick to the plan with more success.

The 5:2 diet is simple to stick to, and is relatively non-invasive. For this reason, it has become a popular "maintenance" regimen, for people who have already tried an Intermittent Fasting plan and would like to return to a more normal eating plan, but at reduced overall calorie intake.

The "Warrior" Diet/Plan

Another plan you're sure to come across in the world of Intermittent Fasting is the Warrior Diet. This has the characteristics of a Diet, rather than a fast, although a major component of the diet is a daily 20 hour Fast, followed by a 4 hour window of large amounts of eating. It refers to "Warriors" like you might refer to our early ancestors, but more modern participants are people who are using Intermittent Fasting to train, cut fat quickly, and focus on muscle building.

The Warrior Diet was designed to take the concept of human evolution-guided eating habits programs another step. The Warrior Diet states that humans are what's known as "nocturnal eaters," which means our species preferred to take our meals after dark. The timing of this consumption is said to lend itself more to the body's natural processes of recovery and rebuilding, which happen most at night during our sleep cycle.

This diet has a lot of food restrictions and guidelines, which make it sound like a version of the Paleo diet. If you've heard of Paleo, you've probably also heard similar messaging about the evolutionary needs of the human diet. The Warrior Diet also allows for small snacks throughout the 20 hour fast period, which are less about calorie consumption and more about keeping your desire to eat occupied without consuming a meal. These snacks might be things like vegetables and nuts, like a prehistoric warrior might find on a long day trek.

Here are some tips for preparing for your first fast:

1. Start with a short fast. Early Dinner, Late Breakfast

The 14/10 fast is almost unnoticeable for most people who are able to sleep 7-8 hours each night. It involves ensuring you are done with dinner by about 7:00 or 7:30PM your first night. Make it a big dinner! Just focus on the food being healthy. Fasting encourages you to get more sleep, since you'll often be using sleep time as fast time. The more you sleep, the easier the fast becomes since your body isn't awake to burn unnecessary energy. When you wake up, resist having breakfast until at least 9:00 or 9:30.

2. Take plenty of liquids

Your body treats hydration differently than it does a large meal. The key is to avoid a large caloric intake during your fast, in order to facilitate your body entering the fast stage. That means that you can have black coffee, water, and tea during your fast. A nice cup of black coffee in the morning might be all you need to keep focused and stay moving! Remember that our bodies are 60% water, and fasting does not mean removing hydration from your routine. If anything, your body needs water more as it ramps up its other processes to support your lack of food.

3. Don't dwell on it

Treat your morning fast as an opportunity to not worry about food. Plan to get something done before your fast ends. Get an errand done, walk the dog, or focus on getting to work a few minutes early to get started. It's incredible what you'll get just by focusing on your own routine instead of eating right away. The important thing is to make good use of that time, so your mind has something to do instead of fixate on food.

4. Don't focus too hard on what time you'll end

One quick way to fail your first fast is to rely too much on your finish line. If you keep telling yourself "I need to make it until 9:30 before I can eat," then your brain will use that as a mantra to become hungrier. Goal setting is a strength of our cognitive process, so let it work against you. Instead, set an activity goal for your fast. Say that you want to get those three things done, then you'll eat.

In this chapter you learned about the primary Intermittent Fasting programs out there, and you learned a few tricks for introducing the fast schedule to your life. In the next chapter, you will learn more about how to exercise while fasting.

5. Stick to it.

It's ok to fail your first few times. It's very hard to introduce change to our routine, especially when that change is to our food consumption processes. This is why dieting can be such a challenging mental process. Just remember that the benefits of fasting accumulate over time. You won't suddenly feel better, or notice your increased vitality and longevity, after one day of fasting. You'll probably experience discomfort for the first week, or the first few days at least. Give your body and your mind time to adapt to the new condition of being hungry. Once you learn what hunger is, beyond just an impulse, you'll start to better understand your body and anticipate its needs.

In this chapter you learned about the primary Intermittent Fasting programs out there, and you learned a few tricks for introducing the fast schedule to your life. In the next chapter, you will learn more about how to exercise while fasting.

Chapter Six
Exercising on a Fast

One of the primary concerns people have when evaluating an Intermittent Fast schedule is where to place a workout. We worry that our workouts need to be precisely timed, even during a full time eating routine, so that we will be at peak energy and exertion to make the workout "worth it." When confronted with the idea of fasting and working out, it's normal to wonder how to support your exercise with proper nutrition.

The most popular way to plan an effective workout is to target late morning. If most fasts are overnight and early morning, then most people on Intermittent Fasts will have time to eat after about noon, until the mid-evening.

Working out can generate a more powerful need to eat in the hours immediately after, so it's important to support that by making sure those urges fit with your fasting plan. A workout at 11:00 AM, ending around noon will place the Intermittent Faster within close reach of a full meal. If, however, you are accustomed to working out early in the morning, before work, then Intermittent Fasting may become difficult to maintain. You will finish your workout and head to the office right as a wave of post-exercise hunger threatens to flatten you. This is a major reason people break their fasts, is when an unexpected hunger pang occurs hours from when the fast is scheduled to end.

Caffeine is a great way to prepare for a fasted workout. Try having a cup of coffee on your way to the gym, knowing that you will be able to eat after you've finished. Before long, your routine will remove any of the lethargy you feel, as your body starts to adapt to the new circumstance and feeds you more of the energy you need. Some experts recommend taking Branch Chain Amino Acids, or "BCAAs," which are taken in liquid form, as helpful supplements to a fasted workout. These amino acids are helpful in synthesizing energy keeping you going during your workout.

A brief word of warning here, especially as you start your workout regimen over a fast. Your body is going to be using different energy stores than it's used to. Instead of the easily accessible sugar stores, your body is most likely in fat burning mode by the time the late morning workout rolls around. Be prepared during your first week to feel different. Stretch appropriately, drink lots more water than you're used to, and give your body time to catch up.

In this brief chapter, you learned more about the strategy for scheduling a workout while fasting. In the next chapters, you will learn what to avoid and what common misconceptions about fasting exist.

Chapter Seven
What to Avoid

In this chapter you will learn about the common mistakes people make in fasting, and how to avoid them.

Long fasts (3 or more days)

Some people might read a short article about Intermittent Fasting, and assume it's the absolute best way to lose weight. The key to losing weight isn't to suddenly stop eating altogether. It isn't a given that the more time you spend in the fast state, the healthier you'll be, the longer you'll live, and the more fit you'll become.

The truth is that your body can enjoy the benefits of the fast state for a certain window of time, and that also needs to be balanced with your comfort level and your ability to fast. You've learned from this book that cognitive abilities don't encounter deterioration even after 48 hours of fasting. But does that mean you should only eat for two days at a time, followed by a two day fast? That doesn't work for most people. Going for two days without food isn't always reasonable.

Further, your body starts to experience deteriorative effects at about 3 days in the fast state. Early in the fast state, your body starts to stimulate hormone production, motivate the usage of fat stores, and focus your mental regeneration. But after 3 days, your body gets more desperate and acts differently. It enters a new type of fast state, one that has the potential to be more dangerous for your well being. Your body begins to sacrifice the integrity of your various systems in order to survive. You certainly won't have much energy on day three, because your body is beginning to shut down. So unless you're Gandhi, you should avoid the long fasts. The book is called "Intermittent" fasting for a reason!

Eating Unhealthy

Another common mistake people make when adopting Intermittent Fasting is similar to mistakes made when a diet introduces a "cheat day." The assumption that whenever a particular program or plan says you "can eat whatever you want" means you can eat poorly in vast volume, is always incorrect.

Intermittent Fasting as a concept does not govern what you eat, just when you eat. But at the end of the day, the most important predictors of our health and wellness are good food, sleep, and regular exercise. There is no method by which the three legs of this "stool" can be cheated, and Intermittent Fasting is no exception.

If you manage to go 24 hours without food, then proceed to consume junk food for 10 hours before resuming your fast, you'll still watch yourself gain weight. Many of the principles of Intermittent Fasting are based on our body's evolutionary abilities, and one of the most powerful abilities we have is the storage of fat for long term survival. Intermittent Fasting may help you access fat burning of these long term stores, but even IF won't help you overcome a bad diet without exercise.

Intermittent Fasting is an opportunity to eat healthier, since you have fewer meals to plan and purchase for. It's not a cure-all for problems of diet and exercise, and it isn't the only thing you need to focus on when crafting a new program.

Fasting When You Shouldn't Be

Fasting isn't right for everyone. Although many people can take advantage of simple fasts like the 14/10, that doesn't mean everyone should try to fast for 24 hours or more.

For example, fasting can affect men and women differently. Women who are pregnant or breastfeeding should avoid longer fasts, since their bodies have different needs during these times. Intermittent fasting, because it is known to stimulate the production of Testosterone and Human Growth

Hormone in both men and women, has been known to affect some women's cycles. Any changes like this to your body should be closely monitored and discussed with a doctor before deciding to continue with a fasting program.

If you have trouble managing your blood sugar, like in cases of Diabetes, then fasting may not be for you. Consult your physician before starting a regimen of Intermittent Fasting if you have been diagnosed with some form of Diabetes.

Children have different nutritional needs, and shouldn't fast excessively.

If you're on some kind of regular medication, be wary of fasting, as food may be a requirement for your prescription.

Intermittent Fasting shouldn't be an excuse to enable an eating disorder. If you're someone who has trouble regulating their food intake, and is prone to excessive binging, then a fast may be setting you up for more of that behavior. Understand the risks, and understand your own body, before deciding whether Intermittent Fasting is for you.

In this chapter, you were given some common mistakes that people make when deciding if fasting is for them. In the next chapter, you'll learn about some of the common misconceptions that are out there about fasting.

Chapter Eight
Common Misconceptions About Fasting

I n this chapter you will learn about some of the common misconceptions that exist about fasting. You will gain the information you need to make more informed decisions about whether fasting is right for you, and what kind of program you should consider.

"I'll just be hungry and irritable"

Not true! Consider the fact that your tendency to become irritable when you haven't eaten is much more a product of your routine than it is a product of your biology. You aren't programmed, after generations of human development, to need to eat every few hours. Your distant ancestors went for days without eating anything, and they survived harsh conditions in order to find food. Your irritability comes from your routine, in which you have taught your body to expect food every few hours. This dependence is easily broken, and can be done gradually with programs like 14/10 and 16/8. This response is mostly mental.

"I won't be able to focus"

This misconception is largely an outgrowth of the first objection. We have trained ourselves to become hungry every few hours, and if we are not fed we become irritable and focus on the perceived need for food. When we are focused on food, and that manifests as a physical hunger, we are setup to become distracted and unfocused. Only after we've broken our modern dependence on a constant need for food and snacking can we release our brains to focus on other things.

"I won't be able to keep up with my fitness goals"

The more we learn about our body's caloric and nutritional requirements, it can seem daunting to make sure that we're providing ourselves the best possible regimen for consuming the correct calories. If we imagine a difficult workout on an empty stomach, we get worried that we'll be lethargic, lacking energy, that we'll be light headed or dizzy.

In reality, these are mental blocks as well. Remember that our bodies actually respond the opposite way to a lack of food. They infuse us with more energy, more focus, and improved cellular processes necessary to help us achieve difficult physical and mental goals because we are in a perceived state of scarcity and need. We are more prone to lethargy after we've eaten, since our body's needs are met.

"Eating more (smaller) meals is what burns fat, not fasting"

There is a common misunderstanding of our body's metabolisms, and it is often compared to the fitness and diet regimens that call for more, smaller meals throughout the day. The worry is that large binge meals are more difficult for our bodies to process, in comparison to small portions spaced throughout the day. It's true that digestion requires a certain amount of energy, and that therefore eating does stimulate your metabolism slightly. But this modest boost in metabolism caused by digestion is small compared to the long term boost to your system from experiencing a fast state at regular intervals. Our bodies haven't spent the majority of their evolutionary careers managing an excess of food, they've been honed to manage calorie deficits. It is a more natural state to take fewer calories over the span of a fasting interval than it is for our bodies to constantly gorge and manage large amounts of calories, and to always be digesting.

Short term fasting has been shown to actually increase your metabolism up to 14%. This is your body kicking into a mode in which it believes you need extra energy to go out and find the next store of food. It is burning fat stores, which require more effort to convert into usable energy, and therefore require a more aggressive metabolic rate to take advantage of.

"Breakfast is the most important meal of the day!"

Most of us grew up hearing this kind of thing all the time. "It's so important!" "It's the only way to start your day!" And finally "It's the best way to get your metabolism going." It's true that eating a meal does raise your metabolism, but only so your body can digest the food you've just given it. If weight loss is your metabolic goal, then reaching the fasted state is probably more beneficial than introducing another load of calories and sugar for your body to focus its efforts on.

Breakfast represents the quickest opportunity for our bodies to experience a productive, Intermittent Fast, since it follows so closely a long period of sleeping fast. Couple with the fact that more than 25% of Americans skip breakfast already, and we can see that there is ample chance for people to take advantage of their body's natural instinct to skip the "most important meal of the day."

"Fasting is just a structured way of starving yourself"

Fasting is not starving. You can eat just as much as you did last week when starting a fast, it is primarily the timing of calorie intake that make fasting different than dieting.

That said, fasting is an early stage of calorie deprivation that eventually becomes starving. The two states are very different, and are characterized by productive bodily processes (fasting) versus the detrimental and deteriorative effects of starving. When fasting, your body is forced to manage the nutrients it has access to more efficiently. Starving forces your body to reach desperately for nutrients in dangerous places, which can put your body at risk of degenerative effects like emaciation.

"I'll lose all my muscle."

Muscle can be difficult to cultivate, so you understandably should be skeptical when being told to limit your caloric intake. Especially when the culture of muscle building seems to focus on constant calorie and protein intake around the clock. It's true, your muscles are always responding to the available protein in your body. But remember that some of the previously unknown effects of Intermittent Fasting include the increased production of Testosterone and the Human Growth Hormone, which are instrumental in creating muscle mass. These are the hormones that professional athletes have been known to cheat in order to use in steroid form, and fasting is a natural way to stimulate production! It's important to pay attention to your protein intake during your eating window, and to make sure that you balance your intake between Whey Proteins and Casein proteins, the longer lasting slow-release proteins that your body can take advantage of many hours later.

Even though you should make sure your body has enough protein to build new muscle, consider the fact that your body won't ever switch to burning your muscle as a source of energy. Your body reserves protein over the long term for your tissues to use, it only really uses Fat and Sugar as a source of energy. You don't have to worry that your body will start consuming your muscles to survive, unless you're many weeks into a fast.

One method thought to further help preserve your protein synthesis during a fast is to consume BCAAs prior to a workout. This will help manage the protein available to your muscles and keep them strong and healthy, preventing potential injury to the musculature.

Intermittent Fasting is probably just another "diet fad."

Intermittent Fasting isn't a diet at all. It's a thoughtful approach to the way we consume calories, not to the specific calories we consume. Intermittent Fasting is an assessment of the vehicle of consumption, rather than the content.

Fasting has been around for centuries, and exists in every corner of the world. Once thought of purely as a religious or spiritual practice, fasting has long thought to offer purification and cleansing properties, in addition to the meditative benefits of this kind of abstention from food and the process of desiring food.

Modern science has just started to examine the evidence supporting Intermittent Fasting, and is weighing that positive evidence with the potentially risky elements of Fasting, those that border on the effects of starvation. In a world burdened by over consumption, the occasional fast is far from our most troubling behavior.

In this chapter you have learnt about some of the common misconceptions when considering whether to incorporate fasting into your diet and exercise plan. If you think fasting might be for you, then the next chapter will help you focus on your first fast!

Chapter Nine
Fasting Around the World

In this chapter you will learn more about the prevalence of fasting around the world. As you begin to understand how widespread fasting is, your confidence in your own abilities will grow. Fasting is often viewed as a practice of purification, which you know understand can be connected to definitive biological evidence.

The Muslim Holy Month of Ramadan

Every year, millions of Muslims around the year observe a Holy Month of Ramadan, during which the faithful will fast from sunrise to sunset each day, and feast at night. This practice has been observed for centuries as a way to purify your body and mind, detach from the material aspects of daily life, pay tribute to God, and pay tribute to the lesser fortunate. From what you've learned so far, a daylight fast doesn't seem so daunting anymore, does it? It is interesting to consider that depending on where you live, your fast as a Muslim may be as long as 20 hours (in places in Scandinavia) or only a few hours (closer to the South Pole).

Early studies on Intermittent Fasting were actually conducted with the consent of Muslims undergoing this regular daily fast, which prohibits the consumption of both food and water while the sun is up. Muslim athletes were interviewed and measured over the course of the month to understand the impact of fasting on the many aspects of physical endurance and mental acuity.

Fasting in the Christian religion

Christians have fasts on their spiritual calendar, but the practice of fasting is positioned in a very similar way: fasting is said to provide focus, a deeper intimacy with God, and can afford penance in this way. Fasting is again viewed as a purification, in direct contrast to the Cardinal sin of Gluttony.

Fasts of Mahatma Gandhi

Mahatma Gandhi made powerful use of fasting as non-violent method of protest and rebellion, and to make moving political statements. Gandhi took 17 fasts, each focused on political and spiritual goals. The longest such fast lasted 21 days.

Fasting Recommended by Benjamin Franklin

Again, primarily as a political and philosophical statement, Benjamin Franklin often warned against the dangers of overeating, and was responsible for promoting the first public fasting day in Philadelphia. He began to record his preference for fasting in one edition of Poor Richard's Almanac, when he wrote that "3 good meals a day is bad living."

Medical Fasting

Have you ever wondered why doctors ask you to fast prior to surgery? The answer has to do with your subconscious. Doctors will be asking your body to slow down everything from breathing to temperature management as they put your under anesthesia, and they don't want your body distracted by trying to digest food during the process. Fasting is also a good way to return your body to accurate levels for measurement.

In the last chapter, you saw more about how fasting has been used the world over as a cultural and political practice.

Final Words

Fasting is making a major modern come back. For centuries, fasting has been a method for purifying the body and achieving heightened states of spirituality and focus. Now, scientific discoveries in the way our bodies process food, produce energy are starting to bring fasting to front pages of major fitness and health blogs around the world.

Fasting takes advantage of our own biology to give our bodies access to the longer term stores of fat to use as energy, instead of relying on a consistent supply of sugar from frequent meals. Beyond weight loss, fasting holds the promise of extended life, better mood, stronger bodies and improved mental acuity. Fasting has been shown to give us access to productive physical and mental states, without any of the deteriorative effects we've feared as a culture for years.

The major obstacle to fasting is mental, it is our own perceived dependence on the regular meal schedule we have come to believe is required for our contentment and health. The key to overcoming this mental barrier is to slowly acclimate our bodies to longer and longer periods of fasting. We only enter the fasted state once 12 hours has passed since our last meal, and only then does our body start to reap the rewards of fasting. At 24 hours, our bodies pass a major threshold from burning sugar for energy to burning fat.

When we fast, we also tap into our bodies' natural ability to heal itself, to regenerate, to become stronger and leaner. We also ask our brains to retain more neurons, a process which has been shown to prevent neurological diseases like Alzheimer's.

By fasting occasionally, we can reduce the time, effort and money spent on food. We can reclaim our meals, to make them celebrations of food and company, rather than the periodic intake of calories. We can be more productive as we take back hours of our day and turn them into focused, dedicated time spent on other things.

Fasting is not the next fad diet. Fasting isn't a diet. It's an approach to food and to our bodies that brings us closer to our biological roots. It's a way to align our lives with the ways our body was designed to operate, rather than the ways society would have us behave. Fasting has been around for centuries and will be around for centuries longer.

It's worth noting that debates around Intermittent Fasting are still very active. Researchers are conducting long term studies that compare the relative benefits of Intermittent Fasting from one routine, like a 16/8 fast, to other routines like 5:2 or periodic 24 hour fasts. Some researchers do not believe at all in the benefits of fasting, and worry instead for people who consider Fasting to be a "quick cure" for any food or weight related issue.

But over the last few years, Intermittent Fasting has certainly gained popularity due to its simplicity and its roots in science and evolution. There is something inherently relatable for many people in the concept of fasting, perhaps because its religious roots stretch far and wide. Our instinct as a people is to use fasting as a way to cleanse our bodies and focus our minds. The science behind fasting can offer us yet another reason for what has become a mainstay in our cultural lives.

If Intermittent Fasting is for you, then good luck! If you aren't sure, consult a doctor before pursuing a new course of diet and fitness. Mention that you're exploring fasting, and you'd like to understand if it's the right course of action for you.

Take care and listen to your body! Enjoy!

www.ingramcontent.com/pod-product-compliance
Lightning Source LLC
Chambersburg PA
CBHW072020290526
45787CB00013B/1521